Evaluating obesity in substitute carers

Mary Mather and
Karen Lehner

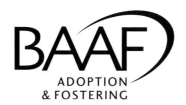

Published by
British Association for Adoption & Fostering (BAAF)
Saffron House
6–10 Kirby Street
London EC1N 8TS
www.baaf.org.uk

Charity registration 275689 (England and Wales) and SC039337 (Scotland)

British Library Cataloguing in Publication Data
A catalogue record for this book is available from the British Library

ISBN 978 1 905664 93 1

Project management by Jo Francis, Publications Department, BAAF
Designed by Helen Joubert Designs
Typeset by Avon DataSet Ltd, Bidford on Avon, Warwickshire B50 4JH
Printed in Great Britain by the Lavenham Press
Trade distribution by Turnaround Publisher Services, Unit 3, Olympia Trading Estate, Coburg Road, London N22 6TZ

BAAF is the leading UK-wide membership organisation for all those concerned with adoption, fostering and child care issues.

Contents

Acknowledgements

We would like to acknowledge the invaluable help of John Simmonds, Director of Policy, Research and Development, Florence Merredew, Health Group Development Officer, and Danielle Sawyer, PA to the Development Team (all at BAAF). We would also like to thank our colleagues on the Health Group Advisory Committee of BAAF as well as health and social care colleagues who made many useful suggestions during consultation.

Note about the authors

This book was written by Dr Mary Mather, Retired Consultant Community Paediatrician, and Dr Karen Lehner, Consultant Community Paediatrician, South West Essex Community Services, Designated Doctor for Looked after Children, South West Essex.

Disclaimer
Earlier drafts of this document were widely circulated during consultation; however, this Good Practice Guide supersedes all previous drafts.

1 Introduction

This good practice guidance was produced at the request of our colleague medical advisers who are increasingly being asked for guidance on obesity by adoption and fostering agencies. It is primarily intended for health and social care professionals who make decisions about the approval of substitute carers and to aid them in matching considerations. It is not a comprehensive guide to the assessment and management of obesity in adults or children, nor will it provide a definitive answer in every case.

Obesity in parents/carers

There are three essential guiding principles in dealing with any difficult health issues in applicants who wish to care for children:

- The welfare of the child is paramount.

- Parenting capacities are more important than perfect health.

- Honesty and openness in dealing with applicants are essential.

We have followed these principles throughout this document. Obesity is a contentious and emotive area of practice, and precise quantification of the health risk which it poses for substitute carers is not possible. This area of practice is always going to involve a judgement based on individual circumstances.

Despite the large amount of research into obesity, when it comes to the substitute care of children there are a number of important unanswered questions. As the percentage of obese adults in Britain continues to increase, the following issues should be the subject of future research.

- Most of the available research on the impact of obesity is based on children living with their birth families. Children come into care with multiple and complex needs in addition to neglected health. There is little data on the additional health impact of living with obese carers.

- The long-term physical and/or psychological impact on a child who is placed with obese

substitute carers is unknown. We have little knowledge about the ways in which substitute carers influence the lifestyle choices of the children placed in their care.

- Parenting is a challenging task. The weight at which obesity significantly limits a person's ability to parent a child is unknown. Research also fails to provide an answer to the very important question of whether an obese adult is still able to provide a healthy environment for a foster or adopted child.

- In the case of kinship care, health factors are often of low secondary consideration. Research does not fully address the importance of health considerations and reduced life expectancy in comparison to the other possible benefits of the placement.

Obesity in looked after children

Anecdotal evidence suggests that obesity in children in the care system is not common. Research into this important area of child health is urgently needed. However, it must be remembered that looked after children often have a complex relationship with food. Looked after children may have been deprived of adequate food as part of a pattern of neglect or as a form of punishment. Many young children come into care with disordered eating patterns, both under- and over-eating. These children are at increased risk of eating disorders in adolescence, because of their high level of unresolved emotional difficulties. It is outside the scope of this guidance to address these issues in detail. Anorexia and bulimia are problems which require specialist psychotherapeutic management. However, both can be preceded by excessive weight gain and low self-esteem, which are features of obesity in adolescents.

Food is also a source of comfort which can be used therapeutically to help children and young people to recover from early traumatic experiences. Food reminds children of their home, their culture, their faith and their lost family relationships. *Recipes for Fostering* (Warman, 2009) explores the relationship between food and fostering through the stories of ten foster carers. These carers share their favourite recipes as well as their experiences of using shopping, cooking and eating together to build relationships with the children they look after.

Any discussion of weight and food with looked after children and young people should be handled with great professional sensitivity. There is little to be achieved in distressing a young person who then refuses to return for any further health guidance. However, it is important to recognise that many children will not be used to a healthy and varied diet and will not have had the opportunity to engage in adequate physical activity. Time, imagination and patience will be needed to support them to adapt as part of the adjustment which comes with entering care. Any adult carers who themselves have had a difficult relationship with food may find it hard to manage this aspect of child care and will need sympathetic support from professionals.

Finally, it should always be remembered that fostered and adopted children are likely to share the physical characteristics and body shape of their birth parents (Stunkard *et al*, 1986) and this information may not be available to future foster carers and adopters. The weight and physical build of birth parents is rarely recorded in social work assessments and is therefore not available to foster carers and adopters.

The British obesity epidemic

In recent years, Britain has become a nation where overweight and obesity in both adults and children are increasingly the norm.

The latest Health Survey for England (HSE) data show that in 2008, 61.4 per cent of adults (aged 16 or over) and 27.3 per cent of children (aged 2–10) in England were overweight or obese; of these, 24.5 per cent of adults and 13.9 per cent of children were obese (Body Mass Index (BMI) greater than 30kg/m2) (Craig *et al*, 2009).

The prevalence of obesity (BMI>30kg/m2) in Scotland has increased over the past two decades, reaching 22 per cent in men and 24 per cent in women in 2003, with marked increases in men aged 35–64 years and in women aged 35–44 years. Obesity in children is now common. In Scotland, nearly one in five (18%) of boys and over one in ten (14%) of girls aged 2–15 years are obese (NHS National Services Scotland, 2009).

In Northern Ireland, the Department of Health and Children (2009) published data on self-reported BMI, showing an increase in obesity of over 30 per cent for both men and women between 1998 and 2007; 59 per cent of men and 41 per cent of women are now self-reporting as either overweight or obese.

By 2050, the Foresight Project (Foresight, 2007) indicated that 60 per cent of adult men, 50 per cent of adult women and about 25 per cent of all children under 16 could be obese. The NHS costs attributable to overweight and obesity are projected to double to £10 billion per year by 2050. The wider costs to society and business are estimated to reach £49.9 billion per year at today's prices. The Foresight Project also predicts that successfully tackling obesity will require a long-term, large scale national commitment. The current prevalence of obesity in the population has been at least 30 years in the making. This will take time to reverse and it is likely to be at least 30 years before reductions in the associated diseases are seen.

Foresight's work indicates that a bold whole-system approach is critical – from production and promotion of healthy diets, to redesigning the environment to promote walking, together with wider cultural changes to shift societal values around food and activity. This will require a broad set of integrated policies including both population and targeted measures and must necessarily include action not only by government, both central and local, but also by society, industry, communities and families as a whole.

As foster carers and adopters are recruited from the general population, which is displaying a trend to increasing body weight, the problem of obesity in substitute carers will not go away. Anecdotal evidence suggests that the problem is increasing. The evidence is also clear that policies aimed solely at individuals will be inadequate and that simply increasing the number or type of small-scale interventions will not be sufficient to reverse this trend. Significant effective action to prevent obesity at a population level is required.

Childhood, adolescence and young adulthood are critical stages in the development of behavioural patterns that will affect children and young people's health in later years. Primary prevention should be the unequivocal first strategy for halting childhood obesity. Statistics from the UK National Child Measurement Programme (2006 07) (DH and DCSF, 2008) indicate the prevalence of overweight/obese children at age 4–5 to be 22.9 per cent. Amongst 10–11-year-old children,

31.6 per cent were overweight/obese. However, the true picture of overweight/obese children may be higher, as these figures were based only on 80 per cent participation and research results indicate that a proportion of children who may be overweight/obese may not have been included in the measurement process. Further emphasising that there is an absolute requirement for an approach to primary prevention of child obesity are the disturbing predictions of the Government's scientific expert committee, the Foresight team, as cited earlier, which predicts that, by 2050, 55 per cent of boys and 70 per cent of girls could be overweight or obese.

The measurement of obesity in adults and children

The National Institute of Clinical Excellence (NICE) (2006) stresses that obesity is a clinical term with health implications and is not concerned with a person's appearance. NICE defines obesity using Body Mass Index (BMI), which is calculated by taking a person's weight in kilograms, divided by their height in metres squared (kg/m2). BMI is categorised by NICE as follows:

Classification	BMI (kg/m²)
Healthy weight	18.5–24.9
Overweight	25–29.9
Obesity I	30–34.9
Obesity II	35–39.9
Obesity III (morbid obesity)	40 or more

Not all obese individuals are at increased risk of cardiovascular disease. However, those with abdominal obesity are at significantly increased risk (Després *et al*, 2001). Waist measurement and waist-to-hip ratio are indicators of a cluster of metabolic abnormalities that increase the risk of cardiovascular disease and diabetes. It is worth identifying these individuals at an early stage so that they have the opportunity to address their increased health risks. A waist measurement greater than 100cm in men and 90cm in women indicates abdominal obesity and the group who are at high risk of future serious health problems (National Heart, Lung and Blood Institute, 1998). The waist-to-hip ratio is worked out by dividing the measurement of the waist (just above the umbilicus) by that of the hips at their widest point.

For men, the ratio should ideally not be over 0.90; for women not over 0.85. The higher the ratio number is above these values, the greater the risk of heart disease.

BMI should be interpreted cautiously in highly muscular individuals, as it is not always a direct measure of body fat. In these individuals, however, the waist-to-hip ratio will be normal. BMI and waist-to-hip ratios can both be calculated quickly and easily using a number of online calculators, such as www.bmi-calculator.net/waist-to-hip-ratio-calculator/.

In children over two years of age, the BMI is a better indicator of overweight or underweight than a weight measurement alone. The new UK/WHO growth charts for children, which include BMI charts, are available online at www.growthcharts.rcpch.ac.uk (Department of Health, 2009). A child whose weight is average for their height will have a BMI between the 25th and 75th centiles, whatever their height centile. A BMI above the 91st centile suggests that the child is overweight. A child with a BMI above the 98th centile is clinically obese.

2 The long-term effects of obesity in adults and children

Obesity is a complex, multi-system disease which not only has a significant impact on physical health, but also on psychosocial wellbeing. Obese people can also experience substantial impairments in their quality of life, including their mental health.

Effects of obesity in adults

The multiple implications of obesity for adults are shown in Figure 1.

Smoking significantly increases all the associated risks of obesity. Current smoking or even having given up smoking in the preceding 12 months significantly increases cardiovascular risk. All overweight and obese individuals must be strongly advised to stop smoking.

The impact of obesity on health is further increased by lack of regular exercise. Obese individuals often lead highly sedentary lifestyles and will need sustained encouragement to change. The Chief Medical Officer (CMO) recommends that adults should achieve a total of at least 30 minutes a day of at least moderate intensity physical activity on five or more days of the week (Department of Health, 2004). This can reduce the risk of cardiovascular disease and type 2 diabetes, and improve psychological wellbeing. The CMO also recommends that for many people, 45–60 minutes of moderate intensity physical activity a day is necessary to prevent obesity. These recommendations are currently under review.

Excessive alcohol intake – the current joint Government recommendations define this as more than 21–28 units per week for men, 14–21 units per week for women (Department of Health, Home Office, Department for Education and Skills and Department for Culture, Media and Sport, 2007) – increases the risk of serious cardiovascular events. Moderate alcohol intake (8 units per week) might decrease it (Lindsay and Hill, 2002).

A family history of premature cardiovascular disease also increases risk. Any applicant whose father or brother suffered a heart attack or died suddenly, at or before the age of 55, or whose mother or sister

suffered a heart attack or died suddenly, at or before the age of 65, is at increased risk.

Men of 45 years and over and women of 55 years and over (or post-menopausal) are also at increased risk of cardiovascular disease (Lindsay and Hill, 2002).

People with any of the following are classified as being at very high risk for disease complications and mortality (over 20 per cent five-year risk of cardiovascular disease):

- established coronary heart disease;
- type 2 diabetes;
- sleep apnoea;
- renal dysfunction;
- familial hypercholesterolaemia or other inherited dyslipidaemias.

Tables have now been devised to quantify more precisely the risk of cardiovascular disease in any individual (British Cardiac Society, British Hyperlipidaemia Association, British Hypertension Society and British Diabetic Association, 2000). They are intended to offer general practitioners reliable advice on the need for lipid-lowering drugs and also to indicate when aggressive treatment of high blood pressure is indicated. (See the information on calculating risk later in this guide.) NICE publishes a range of guidance relevant to assessment of cardiovascular risk factors.

Body shape and size are also closely related to ethnicity. It is well known that the rates of diabetes, hypertension and cardiovascular disease are disproportionately high in certain ethnic groups. However, to exclude people from being adoptive parents or foster carers on the sole criteria of excessive weight and increased cardiovascular risk will leave many children with a limited choice of culturally appropriate substitute carers, is poor practice and could be seen as highly discriminatory. Carers from every minority ethnic group are urgently needed to reflect the increasingly diverse backgrounds of children in the care system.

Figure 1: Medical complications of obesity in adults

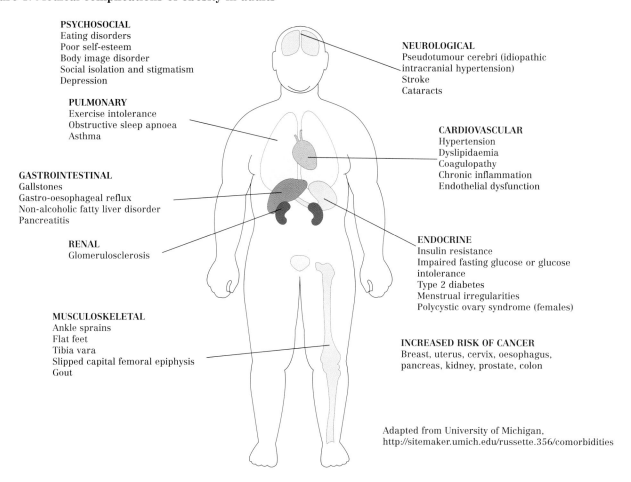

PSYCHOSOCIAL
Eating disorders
Poor self-esteem
Body image disorder
Social isolation and stigmatism
Depression

PULMONARY
Exercise intolerance
Obstructive sleep apnoea
Asthma

GASTROINTESTINAL
Gallstones
Gastro-oesophageal reflux
Non-alcoholic fatty liver disorder
Pancreatitis

RENAL
Glomerulosclerosis

MUSCULOSKELETAL
Ankle sprains
Flat feet
Tibia vara
Slipped capital femoral epiphysis
Gout

NEUROLOGICAL
Pseudotumour cerebri (idiopathic intracranial hypertension)
Stroke
Cataracts

CARDIOVASCULAR
Hypertension
Dyslipidaemia
Coagulopathy
Chronic inflammation
Endothelial dysfunction

ENDOCRINE
Insulin resistance
Impaired fasting glucose or glucose intolerance
Type 2 diabetes
Menstrual irregularities
Polycystic ovary syndrome (females)

INCREASED RISK OF CANCER
Breast, uterus, cervix, oesophagus, pancreas, kidney, prostate, colon

Adapted from University of Michigan,
http://sitemaker.umich.edu/russette.356/comorbidities

Glossary

Obstructive sleep apnoea: intervals when an individual stops breathing while they are asleep
Gastro-oesophageal reflux: stomach contents move back up into the oesophagus (tube leading from mouth to stomach) causing a burning sensation, pain and long-term damage to the lining of the oesophagus.
Pancreatitis: inflammation of the pancreas which causes abdominal pain and disrupts liver functioning
Glomerulosclerosis: degenerative disorder of the kidneys impairing their functioning.
Tibia vara: a bowing of the lower legs
Slipped capital femoral epiphysis: the head of the femur/thigh bone slips out of normal alignment at the growing point of the bone.
Dyslipidaemia: abnormal levels of fats/lipids in the blood, including hypercholesterolemia/high cholesterol and high triclycerides.
Coagulopathy: abnormality of clotting factors in the blood.
Endothelial dysfunction: abnormality of the tissue layer lining the blood vessels.

Effects of obesity in children

Extensive research has taken place into the implications of obesity in adults, but there is less information about the effects of obesity in children, as this is a relatively new area of paediatric practice. However, obesity in children is associated with a number of increased risks, as shown in Figure 2.

Wake *et al* (2008) systematically reviewed the other consequences of obesity in Australian children. These included the following.

• Overweight and obese school-aged children may experience more daytime tiredness, snoring, less night-time sleep and more injury-related morbidity than non-overweight children.

- Obese, but not overweight, children were 72 per cent more likely to have additional health care needs compared with non-overweight children, in particular an increased tendency to asthma.

- Parents of overweight/obese pre-school children reported relatively few additional health burdens over and above those of the non-overweight pre-schoolers. Parents were more likely to be concerned about sleep, respiratory problems and school readiness. These findings may shed light on the disparity between strong public concern and parental lack of concern about overweight/obesity at school entry.

- This study also suggests that interventions that reduce overweight/obesity present at school entry have the potential to prevent the later onset of childhood morbidities associated with obesity.

Social workers, adopters and foster carers may similarly be more concerned about issues such as attachment, learning and behaviour rather than a child's weight. They could therefore miss a valuable opportunity to address this issue at an early stage and decrease the risk of long-term health problems.

Obese children appear more likely to experience psychological or psychiatric problems than children of normal weight. Obesity could make a child more reluctant to take part in physical exercise and exposes them to increased risks of bullying from other children (Rees *et al*, 2009).

In addition to the risks detailed above, in the short term, paediatric obesity has been associated with

Figure 2: Medical complications of obesity in children

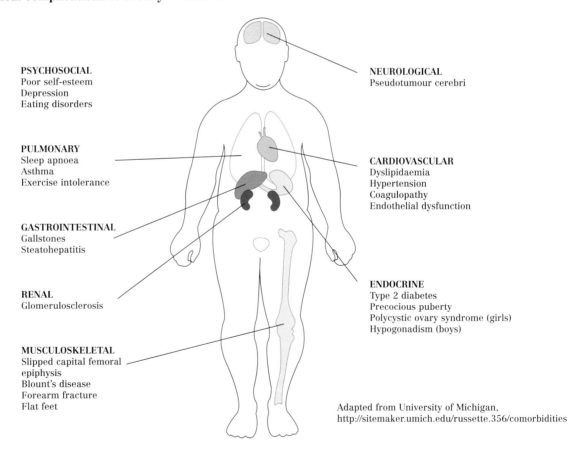

PSYCHOSOCIAL
Poor self-esteem
Depression
Eating disorders

PULMONARY
Sleep apnoea
Asthma
Exercise intolerance

GASTROINTESTINAL
Gallstones
Steatohepatitis

RENAL
Glomerulosclerosis

MUSCULOSKELETAL
Slipped capital femoral epiphysis
Blount's disease
Forearm fracture
Flat feet

NEUROLOGICAL
Pseudotumour cerebri

CARDIOVASCULAR
Dyslipidaemia
Hypertension
Coagulopathy
Endothelial dysfunction

ENDOCRINE
Type 2 diabetes
Precocious puberty
Polycystic ovary syndrome (girls)
Hypogonadism (boys)

Adapted from University of Michigan,
http://sitemaker.umich.edu/russette.356/comorbidities

Glossary

Steatohepatitis: accumulation of fat in the liver, accompanied by inflammation.

Blount's disease: progressive bowing of the lower legs, thought to be due to the effects of weight on the growth plate. The condition is more common among children of African ancestry.

liver disease, cardiovascular risk factors, asthma, diabetes (types 1 and 2) and orthopaedic abnormalities (Reilly and Wilson, 2006).

Evidence linking childhood obesity to adult disease and premature mortality is difficult to obtain and is currently limited. However, systematic review and critical appraisal are supportive of the hypothesis that paediatric obesity has adverse effects on health in childhood and that, unless corrected, these problems will continue into adolescence and adult life (Reilly and Wilson, 2006).

Clearly, the increasing prevalence of obesity in childhood is very likely to translate into greatly increased levels of obesity among adults, rendering them more susceptible to chronic life-threatening illness. The trend of weight problems in children is a particular cause for concern because of evidence suggesting a "conveyor-belt" effect in which excess weight in childhood continues into adulthood. A US study found that 55 per cent of obese 6–9-year-olds and 79 per cent of obese 10–14-year-olds remained obese into adulthood (Cross-Government Obesity Unit, Department of Health and Department for Children, Schools and Families, 2009).

3 Principles for dealing with applicants to adopt or foster

General principles concerning health assessment

The final decision regarding the approval of adopters and foster carers is not a medical one. It is ultimately made by the agency decision-maker on the recommendation of adoption and fostering panels. Although health information is important, it is not the sole criterion on which panel recommendations should be made. Medical reports are given to panels to assist in the approval and matching of prospective parents with vulnerable children. They must not be used to exclude all but the very fit. It is absolutely essential that the agency medical adviser does not see their role as one of accepting or rejecting a particular applicant purely on health grounds. It is important that doctors and social workers should not use evidence about one health issue to reject applicants where there is a range of issues of concern.

As previously stated, there are three guiding principles in dealing with difficult health issues in applicants:

- The welfare of the child is paramount.

- Parenting capacities are more important than perfect health.

- Honesty and openness in dealing with applicants are essential.

Parenting involves more than good health. It requires evidence of a prospective parent's or carer's values, attitudes, life experiences, commitment and flexibility in responding to the needs of individual children.

If initial medical information raises serious concerns, agencies should consider an early health/social care discussion about any contentious health issues. Full health assessment at an early stage, supplemented with the advice of the medical adviser, can be extremely useful for social workers, highlighting areas where the panel will require further information when the case returns for the final recommendation. However, for adoption cases in England, these medical assessments must be conducted within the formal assessment process, so that applicants can access their right to independent review by approaching the Independent Review Mechanism (IRM) where

applicable (Adoption and Children Act 2002, Guidance 2005 Chapter 3, paras 52–57). In Wales the Independent Review Mechanism Cymru can provide independent review. In Northern Ireland, the Adoption Policy and Procedures currently require that health checks are part of the preliminary checks undertaken prior to the preparation course. Serious health concerns are still discussed at the panel at an early stage in relation to taking panel advice on whether a full assessment should be undertaken at that time. In fostering situations, while it is not stipulated that health checks are undertaken before the preparation course, it is relatively common practice to seek early advice from the panel where there are serious health concerns. While there is no statutory IRM process, there is a process for reviewing panel recommendations and the decision-maker's decision. In Scotland, the position is much the same as it is in Northern Ireland and while there is no IRM, there are provisions for reviewing agency decisions about prospective carers.

When applying to adopt or foster, all applicants need to have a comprehensive health assessment, undertaken by their general practitioner. In cases of serious illness, it is essential to obtain additional written permission to approach any specialists who have been responsible for the patient's care. It is advisable to ask the consultant, in writing, very specific questions including the impact of the condition on daily functioning, the short- and long-term prognosis and the chance of a prolonged period of debilitating illness. It is also important to ensure that the consultant understands the need for robust physical and mental health to parent a child with complex needs, and the need for applicants to have a reasonable probability of being able to parent a child until adulthood. Morbid obesity, given the well-established long-term risks of this condition, must be considered as a health factor which could cause serious long-term illness and premature death in an applicant.

Medical advisers and social workers need to remember that adults whose application is turned down by an agency have a right to know on what grounds they were rejected. Hence, doctors and social workers should be scrupulously open and honest from the beginning.

It must always be remembered that in most cases it is a couple, not an individual, who come forward to be considered as carers. Social workers and medical advisers need to carefully consider the illogical situation of rejecting a healthy, well-motivated applicant because of health problems in their partner. Where one applicant has significant health risks, the assessment must focus on the motivation and abilities of both partners and their support networks. The social worker will need to weigh up the potential impact of declining health in one partner on the capacity of the other to cope with their partner's illness. There will also be an unpredictable impact on the carer's birth children and any other children in placement, which needs to be carefully considered.

Practitioners also need to evaluate the impact of possible premature parental death on children and young people who have already experienced significant losses. The conclusion might still be that the possible benefits to the child of lifetime family membership in a matched placement outweigh the overall risk.

The aim of substitute care is to provide needy children with nurturing carers and secure, stable placements which last as long as the child needs them. It is illogical to have health standards which are based solely on the estimated length of the placement: short-term foster placements frequently become long-term by default. Medical advisers and agencies should apply the same health standards for foster carers and adopters.

Health standards for kinship carers, where different standards are often applied, are currently an issue of concern for medical advisers. In 2004–05, a large study of 113 kinship placements made between 1995 and 2001 were examined in depth (Hunt *et al*, 2008). Concerns about the health of carers were identified in 22 cases at the time of care proceedings. These included diabetes, arthritis, stroke, previous heart attack, cancer, dementia, and psychiatric and degenerative disease in either the applicant or their partners. In this medium-term follow-up study, however, only one placement had broken down because of ill-health.

Difficult decisions and dilemmas about adult health must always be balanced against the large numbers of waiting children, particularly older children, sibling groups, black and minority ethnic children and children with other special needs. Whilst it is

important to try to prevent the premature disruption of a placement because of illness or death, the quality of family life will always be more important to a child than the physical health of his or her carers.

4 Specific issues concerning obesity in substitute carers

There are currently no national guidelines regarding obesity in adoptive parents, foster carers, or kinship carers. The authors believe that this should be addressed by both health and social services, as all the available evidence suggests that the issue of obesity will only get worse. As an applicant's BMI increases, there is an increasing risk of health complications. Every opportunity, whether at assessment or annual review, should be taken to promote healthy lifestyles in the interests of the applicant and their family. This is particularly pertinent when the weight of a valued carer is increasing over time.

National UK guidance emphasises the importance of health promotion awareness for foster carers, both in relation to their own health and that of children in their care (*National Minimum Standards for Fostering Services in England*[1] (Department of Health, 2002) and Wales (2003), the *National Standards for Foster Care* for Northern Ireland (Department for Health and Children, 1999) and the *National Care Standards Foster Care and Family Placement Services* for Scotland (Scottish Executive, 2005).

We fully acknowledge that many excellent substitute carers are obese. There is also a UK-wide shortage of both foster carers and adopters. We also recognise that the risk of placing a child in a household where one or more of the adults is obese is only one factor in the complex process of the holistic assessment of a child's needs. We are also mindful of the importance of not disrupting stable placements which are otherwise meeting the needs of a child. However, it is the responsibility of the placing agency to ensure that any health risks to the child are identified, brought to the attention of their carers, and measures put in place to reduce the impact of the problem.

Agencies also have a primary responsibility to ensure that where relationships are established between a child and a carer, these are maintained for as long as the child needs them. It is a tragedy for a child who has already experienced significant losses to then lose a foster, adoptive or kinship carer because of preventable illness or premature death.

Adoption agencies have to take into account that it is not helpful to impose "blanket" bans when considering applications from prospective adopters. The issue is not therefore one of banning prospective carers, but of engaging with them, and providing information, advice and education about healthy diets and active lifestyles.

All recent Government publications in this area emphasise the importance of securing optimum health for looked after children (*Care Matters: Transforming the lives of children and young people in care* (in England) (Department for Education and Skills, 2006); *Care Matters: A bridge to a better future* (in Northern Ireland) (Department of Health, Social Services and Public Safety, 2007); *Looked After Children and Young People: We can and must do better* (in Scotland) (Scottish Executive, 2007); and *Children and Young People: Rights to Action* (in Wales) (Welsh Assembly Government, 2004)).

Care Matters expresses this duty in a powerful way:

> *As the corporate parent of children in care, the State has a special responsibility for their wellbeing. Like any good parent, it should put its own children first. That means being a powerful advocate for them to receive the best of everything and helping children to make a success of their lives.*

As the problem of obesity in the UK increases, agencies will have to balance the positive elements of any placement against the negative health impact of a family environment which encourages obesity. Starting now to address the importance of healthy lifestyles in all the families of looked after children will not only protect the long-term health of our children and their carers, but also reduce potential problems for agencies in the future.

---

[1] Subject to current revision.

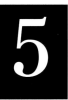

5 Recommendations to social workers and panel members

The recommendation about whether to approve an obese applicant to adopt or foster should never be delegated to the medical adviser. This must always be a joint recommendation in which social workers and panel members have an important role.

The applicant's health assessment by the general practitioner is an invaluable opportunity for a comprehensive health review. It offers applicants an opportunity to re-evaluate their lifestyle and for the general practitioner to recommend intervention which offers positive long-term benefits. Most agencies will have encountered applicants whose undiagnosed hypertension or diabetes was first picked up during a routine medical examination.

Obese individuals frequently suffer from social stigmatisation and discrimination and the relevance of obesity to the health assessment of prospective carers is inevitably controversial. It is, however, paramount that the assessing social worker raises any concerns about weight with applicants during the information and advice stage, and advises them that obesity will be an issue for the panel to consider. As with any identified issue, it is always advisable to have a health assessment early in the assessment process, followed by a discussion with the medical adviser. The applicant should also be advised by the assessing social worker that the medical adviser will want to write to their general practitioner and that they may have to have further investigations. It is important that any medical information which causes concern to the worker is addressed during the assessment process before being presented to the panel.

The following important factors will not necessarily emerge during a routine medical examination, but must be evaluated and evidenced by the social worker prior to any recommendation.

- What is the applicant's understanding of the causes of obesity and how it contributes to ill health?

- What is the applicant's understanding of a healthy diet for their family? Are any other family members overweight or obese? Have previous children placed with this applicant gained excessive weight?

- What is their attitude to physical activity, both for themselves and any children placed with them? What is their capacity to engage in physical activity? Do they become breathless climbing one flight of stairs? Could they chase a toddler who runs towards a road?

- Are these applicants able to provide a child with at least 60 minutes or more of physical activity every day? If carers are prevented from accessing a range of physical activities for the child because there are too many children in the placement or because of numerous professional meetings, attending hospital appointments or contact arrangements, the agency should consider whether, as the corporate parent, they are doing everything possible to maximise the life chances of looked after children.

- Does the applicant want to lose weight? Successful weight loss depends very largely on motivation. An unmotivated applicant is unlikely to lose weight. Their previous history of successful and unsuccessful weight loss attempts is important.

- Does the applicant have the time and/or resources to achieve successful weight loss? Is the applicant's general practitioner supportive? Has he or she offered appropriate interventions?

Professionals who are themselves overweight might have difficulties dealing with these issues in a dispassionate way. However, they should prioritise the present and future health of the applicants and the welfare of the children in their professional practice in this area.

The conclusions of this analysis should be recorded by the assessing worker and made available to any matching panel or at future reviews, where appropriate.

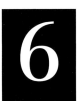

6 Recommendations to children's services and placement agencies

Agencies should set in place a long-term strategic framework to ensure that the recognised health risks and consequences of obesity in parents, carers and children are incorporated into routine practice and decision-making. They need to become more aware of the importance of training all social workers in these issues.

- The importance of a healthy lifestyle, diet and exercise should be included in all initial training for prospective foster carers and adopters. These discussions should be ongoing throughout the approval and review process. Agencies should also provide regular training and information on the health implications of obesity for fostering, adoption and permanency panels.

- The importance and constituents of a healthy lifestyle should be discussed at all household reviews. This is especially important where either a carer has an elevated BMI or if a child is gaining excessive weight in the placement. Where both birth parents are overweight or obese, a child is six times more likely to be overweight or obese than a child who has birth parents of a healthy weight (Cross-Government Obesity Unit, Department of Health and Department for Children, Schools and Families, 2009).

- Carers, residential home staff and social workers should be advised not to use unhealthy food as a reward or pacifier for children and young people, especially those with behaviour difficulties.

- Social workers should not entertain children and young people in care at venues where fast food and food high in sugar, fat and salt are the only available option.

- Local authorities should ensure that the quality of food in residential homes is nutritionally adequate for the needs of growing children.

- All local authorities should make available free or reduced price leisure activities for looked after children and their "host" families, to encourage physical activity.

- In kinship placements, which are of particular concern to medical advisers, the additional health risks to the child of being placed in a household where there are carers who are overweight or obese need to be carefully balanced against the other benefits of the placement for the child.

7 Recommendations to medical advisers

The role of the medical adviser in the assessment of adult applicants

An informal survey of 52 medical advisers in 2009 showed that 96 per cent of those surveyed would like guidance on obesity because they considered that the problem was increasing. Although 61 per cent had had serious medical concerns about obese applicants, these concerns were nearly always discounted by social workers and panel members. There was general agreement that any guidance for health practitioners should take into account the level of obesity in adult applicants, and the presence or absence of complications.

Whilst few doctors thought that BMI alone should be the sole criteria for assessment, there was a consensus that, as BMI increases, a cut-off point should be considered such that an application might be deferred.

Applicants who are overweight (BMI 25 to 30 kg/m²)

As an applicant's BMI increases, there is an increasing risk of health complications. Every opportunity, whether at assessment or annual review, should be taken to promote healthy lifestyles in the interest of the applicant and their family. This is particularly pertinent when the weight of a valued carer is increasing over time. Applicants should be made aware of the increased risks of smoking if they are overweight. They also need to appreciate the increased risk of diabetes, high blood pressure and other health complications.

Applicants who are obese (BMI 30 to 40 kg/m²)

Waist measurement or waist-to-hip ratio as recorded on the BAAF Form AH should be used to identify applicants who are at high risk of obesity-related complications. A waist measurement of more than 100cm in a man and 90cm in a woman increases cardiovascular risk 20-fold, even in the absence of other complications (National Heart, Lung and Blood Institute, 1998). Applicants who fall into this category need to be made aware that they have a particularly high-risk form of obesity.

Medical advisers should alert applicants and their general practitioners to the presence of other health factors identified on Form AH, for example, cigarette smoking, hypertension, high cholesterol, diabetes, family history of cardiovascular disease, which could increase the risk of further morbidity and mortality. Treatment of these health issues could offer significant positive health benefits even without weight loss. Jackson (2000) notes that any reduction of risk factors will lessen the risk of cardiovascular disease, whether or not efforts at weight loss are successful.

Applicants should be advised to visit their primary health care team to discuss their weight. It would be good practice for medical advisers to have standard letters to social workers which are also copied to the applicants and their general practitioner. Any comments about weight and health must be tactful and sensitive to the distress which might result. Where further investigations are needed, they should be initiated in the spirit of promoting the health of the applicant, rather than excluding them from further assessment or approval. Treatment options for consideration will depend upon the individual and their own doctor's advice, but may include dietary changes, increasing physical activity, behaviour modification and drug therapy.

In cases where applicants or their general practitioners fail to take action, social workers, approval and matching panels will have to balance the potential health implications for the carer and the child against the other benefits of the placement.

Applicants who are morbidly obese (BMI over 40 kg/m²)

NICE (2006) has identified obesity at this level as a very serious health problem that cannot be ignored as part of an assessment. This group of applicants is at high risk of significant morbidity and early mortality, which could impact on their ability to care for a child. In order to reach a fair and balanced decision about applicants who fall into this category, it is essential that the following information is available to the medical adviser:

- accurate family history with ages and causes of death in first degree relatives (parents, full siblings and children);

- the results of relevant investigations, for example, diabetes, fasting blood sugar, pre-treatment cholesterol, accurate blood pressure: this will enable a cardiovascular risk to be calculated using one of the available online resources;

- accurate lifestyle information, particularly concerning smoking and alcohol;

- whether other family members, particularly other children in the family, are either overweight or obese;

- information on the applicant's understanding of the risks of their medical condition, and their motivation and attitude to change.

Some of this information will be obtained from the general practitioner, some from the applicant's Form AH and some from a thorough home-based assessment by the social worker.

It is good practice for the medical adviser to refer an applicant with this degree of obesity back to their general practitioner in the expectation that the general practitioner will follow the NICE guidelines or their equivalent and, where necessary, refer the applicant for specialist local services. This may well include consideration for medical and/or surgical treatment.

For applicants in this category, the final decision about the application must be made on an individual basis following a multi-agency discussion, and be sensitive to the feelings of the applicant and the needs of children needing placement. Agencies must appreciate that morbid obesity with complications is a very serious medical condition which might not be compatible with the physical and emotional challenges of substitute parenting.

Calculating risk

Medical advisers must make risk assessments on sound evidence rather than on prejudice. Risk predictions must also be interpreted in the light of any

lifestyle changes that are put into place, for instance, stopping smoking or the successful treatment of hypertension or high cholesterol. All these interventions will significantly reduce morbidity and mortality and offer positive health benefits (see the case examples later in this chapter for more details).

There are now a number of online calculation tools which calculate the risk of an individual having a heart attack or stroke in the next ten years. None include all the known risk factors, but they are useful for presenting a large amount of complex information in a form which applicants and panels can easily understand. However, these tools can only provide guidance in the context of all the information obtained through a comprehensive health and social care assessment.

As part of the Quality and Outcomes Framework for general practice (General Medical Services Contract), (NHS, 2004), all general practitioners in England, Scotland and Wales now undertake cardiovascular risk assessments in any patient over 40. Any patient under the age of 40 is entitled to ask their general practitioner to do a risk assessment as part of a well-person check. The information should therefore be readily available for medical advisers to access. Most general practitioners in England and Wales use the QRISK®2-2010 risk calculator, available at www.qrisk.org. To use this tool requires knowledge of an individual's age, sex, ethnicity, family history in first-degree relatives, BMI, systolic blood pressure, cholesterol/HDL ratio, smoking history and whether they have diabetes, chronic kidney disease or rheumatoid arthritis. It is not suitable for people who already have a diagnosis of heart disease or stroke. ASSIGN is the cardiovascular risk score chosen for use in Scotland, available at www.assign-score.com, and which includes social deprivation as well as other risk factors. Practitioners in Northern Ireland utilise a variety of measurement tools to assess cardiovascular risk.

Figure 3 shows the QRISK®2-2010 risk assessment tool. Whilst this is not a perfect tool, it does provide some useful data to guide decision making.

Using the QRISK®2-2010 tool

Example 1

Helen is a 32-year-old woman who has had two renal transplants. She has a stable seven-year marriage, a supportive partner and her family live locally. Her husband is a 38-year-old teacher, who is at home in the school holidays. He is fit and well. Helen is a

Figure 3: QRISK®2-2010 cardiovascular disease risk calculator

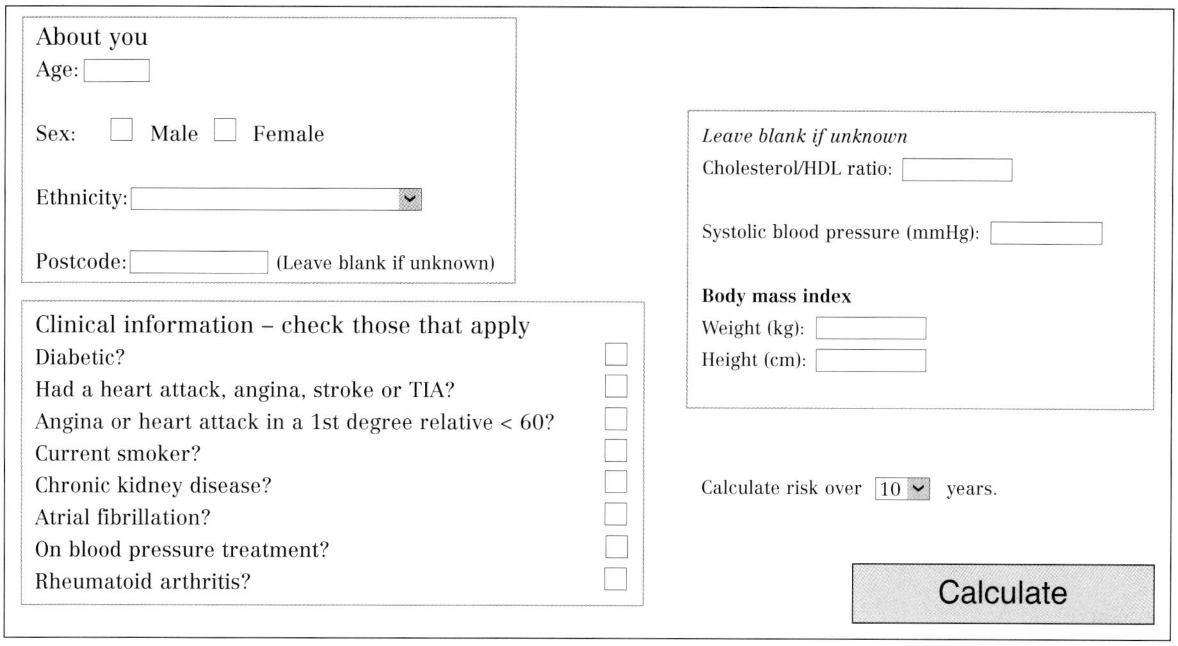

Reproduced with kind permission from Julia Hippisley-Cox, University of Nottingham. Copyright © 2008-10 Julia Hippisley-Cox, University of Nottingham

registered childminder with an outstanding Ofsted inspection. She and her husband wish to adopt a six-year-old boy.

The following factors need to be considered and can be put into the risk tool:

a) Helen is on medication for high blood pressure, but this controls her blood pressure well. The last recording was 130/70.
b) She has no family history of heart disease.
c) Her BMI is 23, with a waist measurement of 62cm.
d) She is a non-smoker.
e) Her creatinine (used as a measurement of renal function) is stable at 214 and her blood glucose is 4.5.
f) Her cholesterol is 5, HDL 1.3, LDL 2.6.

Using the QRISK®2-2010 risk calculation tool shows her to have a risk of developing heart disease or having a stroke during the next 10 years of less than 10 per cent.

Example 2

Limited information is available about Hasan, a 39-year-old Bangladeshi who wishes to offer permanency to his seven-year-old orphan nephew.

The following factors need to be considered and can be put into the risk tool:

a) Hasan has a family history of early onset heart disease: his father died at the age of 48 of a heart attack.
b) He is a smoker.
c) He is overweight with a BMI of 37.5.
d) He is on treatment for hypertension with a current blood pressure of 145/90.
e) His lipids and blood sugar are unknown.

Using the QRISK®2-2010 risk calculation tool shows him to have a risk of developing heart disease or having a stroke during the next 10 years of 36 per cent.

• The score for a typical person with the same age, sex and ethnicity without Hasan's risk factors is only 2 per cent.

• Stopping smoking would reduce his risk to 21 per cent.

• Reducing his BMI to 31 by diet and exercise would reduce his risk to 18 per cent.

• Improving his blood pressure control would reduce the risk to 14 per cent.

Given his very high QRISK®2 score, Hasan urgently needs this information to protect himself and his family. These measures can all be addressed as part of his application. To exclude Hasan on the sole criterion of his increased cardiovascular risk will deprive his nephew of the opportunity to grow up within his birth family and culture, which would be both discriminatory and poor practice. Hasan's application is an ideal chance to improve his life expectancy, at the same time as offering his nephew the opportunity to find permanence and security.

The QRISK®2-2010 tool also shows the importance of knowing an applicant's ethnic background. The following table shows the 10-year risk of developing heart disease for different ethnicities, keeping all other risk factors the same as in Example 2 above.

Ethnicity	10-year risk of developing heart disease or having a stroke
Bangladeshi	36%
Indian	27%
White	21%
Chinese	15%
Black African	14%

The role of the medical adviser with looked after children

All children and young people in care in the UK must have a statutory health assessment carried out at specified intervals. We strongly recommend that this assessment should always include a calculation of BMI in all children over two years of age. This must then be plotted on the new UK/WHO growth charts for children, available at www.growthcharts.rcpch.ac.uk. These charts are essential in the assessment of all children and must be used by all medical advisers and specialist nurses. Children with a BMI above the 91st centile are considered to be overweight, and children above the 98th centile are considered to be obese. The medical adviser or specialist nurse should bring the situation to the attention of the foster carer, social worker and, where appropriate, the child or young person.

It should be borne in mind that the BMI may occasionally give misleading results in children who have a very muscular build, especially boys. It is well known, for example, that some athletes, especially in strength sports, have high BMIs but low levels of body fat. If there is any doubt, a waist measurement should also be plotted on a standard reference chart. The waist measurement in muscular children will be within normal parameters. However, the routine measurement of waist size is not recommended in children.

For children in the care system who already experience considerable disadvantage, becoming obese in childhood could add to the well-recognised physical and mental heath problems they might face as adults. Detailed guidance on the management of obesity in childhood is available from NICE (2006), and all medical advisers and specialist nurses for looked after children should be familiar with, or may find it useful to consult, this evidence-based report. Health professionals in England should also be familiar with the statutory guidance, *Promoting the Health and Well Being of Looked after Children* (Department for Children, Schools and Families, and Department of Health, 2009), which contains advice on both diet and activity specifically for children in the care system and their carers. Paediatricians might also be interested in consulting Baumer's review article (2007).

Young people with a BMI over 40 should be referred initially to their general practitioner or to local paediatric services for further assessment. The cornerstone of treatment involves lifestyle changes, including improved eating patterns and increased exercise. Drug treatment is not generally recommended for children under the age of 12 years. For children aged 12 and over, such treatment should be started only by a specialist team. Surgical intervention is not generally recommended in children or young people. Bariatric surgery (surgery to assist weight loss) may be considered for young people only in exceptional circumstances, and if they have achieved or nearly achieved physiological maturity (NICE, 2006).

Case examples

Placing children in a family where there are significant health risks in either partner needs to be weighed up against the specific advantages of the placement. It is very important that the medical adviser and the assessing social work team liaise closely wherever there are serious health concerns. The following case examples are composites from the many cases seen by the authors and illustrate some of the common practice dilemmas. These cases are not meant to provide the definitive answer to case management, but are intended as examples of good multi-disciplinary working in complex cases where health and social care have a role to play, and where the interest of the child is paramount. The dilemmas we have chosen have been selected by our medical colleagues as examples of the common problems which they regularly experience.

Frequently, medical advisers have only the information provided on the adult health Form AH. They are often expected to make recommendations in the absence of any knowledge of the other strengths of the applicant or the needs of the specific child.

1. A kinship carer

Dr A receives Form AH on Mrs L. The applicant is a 55-year-old black African single carer with a BMI of 41.5. She is a non-smoker who is on treatment for high blood pressure, with a systolic blood pressure of 145mm Hg. She is diabetic and has a past history of treatment for early breast cancer 10 years ago. Using the QRISK®2-2010 calculation tool, her risk of developing heart disease during the next 10 years is 9 per cent.

Dr A subsequently questions whether the application should be approved on medical grounds, but is then informed by the social worker that the child in question is Mrs L's four-year-old grandson, who has been living with her for 10 months.

The doctor and social worker must liaise to consider the relative balance of risk. Mrs L is at risk of further serious medical problems in the future, but this risk must be weighed against the advantages of a family placement and the potential harm to her grandson of moving after a year's stability. If the placement goes ahead, the support package provided by the local authority should be robust and must always include contingency planning for adverse health outcomes in the future.

The following actions should be taken:

- The medical adviser should write to the applicant's GP (copying the letter to Mrs L), requesting a review of her general health. This should include ensuring that she has optimal control of her blood pressure and consideration of the NICE guidelines for management of her obesity. In this letter, it would be helpful for the medical adviser to explain the reason for the

request and the importance of good health in Mrs L's ability to provide long-term care for a very young child.

- Mrs L should give written consent for the medical adviser to write to her consultant oncologist about the prognosis for her breast cancer.

- Mrs L may not have access to advice on good nutrition. The health visitor and/or practice nurse should be asked to advise Mrs L about appropriate diet and physical activity for herself and the child.

- The local authority should assess in what other ways Mrs L and her grandson could be supported, given the increased health risks in this placement. They should explore whether other family members can provide appropriate exercise opportunities for the little boy if Mrs L is unable to do this. Free local authority leisure centre passes will encourage physical activity for them both.

- Is Mrs L receiving sufficient financial support to provide a healthy diet? The local authority should ensure that the financial support is adequate to enable Mrs L to provide this.

- The care plan will need to ensure that other friends/family members develop a relationship with the child in case Mrs L becomes ill and alternative care is needed.

- Careful consideration must be given to legal planning and the most appropriate placement orders to protect her grandson if Mrs L becomes ill or dies during his childhood. Mrs L can nominate a legal guardian in her will, but only if she has parental responsibility. She cannot do this as a foster carer.

2. A specific adoption application

It is a recognised fact of modern adoption practice that applicants with serious health risks are rarely approved as adopters for babies and very young children, as there are many other alternative healthy carers available. However, adopters with serious health problems are often considered for "difficult to place" young children with complex needs. Medical advisers struggle with these cases. They are often under considerable pressure to recommend the applicants as no other prospective adopters have come forward but are aware that, in doing so, a vulnerable child is at increased risk of losing a parent because of increasing disability or early death. This risk must be balanced against the potential harm to a young child of growing up in the care system, and loss of the opportunity to grow up in a positive family environment.

J is a six-year-old child of dual white and Asian heritage with a diagnosis of severe learning difficulties and an autistic spectrum disorder. He has been in care since the age of two years. Following local publicity as part of National Adoption Week, Mr and Mrs W expressed interest in becoming his adopters. They have a stable 10-year marriage and two birth children, one of whom has a mild autistic spectrum disorder. Mrs W is Indian and her husband is white. They have been local authority foster carers in England for 10 years and have outstanding references. They have good links with the local branch of the National Autistic Society and their own child, despite his difficulties, is doing very well.

Mrs W is 50 and morbidly obese with a BMI of 45. She has been on medication for high blood pressure for 15 years with a systolic blood pressure of 140mm Hg. Following a hysterectomy two years ago, she spent three weeks in intensive care with a pulmonary embolus (a life-threatening blood clot in the lungs and a well recognised post-operative complication associated with obesity). Using the QRISK®2-2010 calculation tool, her risk of developing heart disease during the next 10 years is 7 per cent. Mr W is 52 and is a newly diagnosed type 2 diabetic. He is also obese with a BMI of 36. Using the QRISK®2-2010 tool, his risk of developing heart disease during the next 10 years is 13 per cent. Both are non-smokers.

The agency medical adviser is very concerned about the fact that both applicants have potentially life-shortening chronic disorders, and recommended to the panel that the application should be turned down on medical grounds. The social worker was very keen to approve the application. The panel, however, agreed with the medical adviser and voted against the placement. The decision-maker supported the panel recommendation. The couple took their case to the Independent Review Mechanism,[2] which found in favour of the couple.

---

2 Independent Review Mechanism in England, Independent Review Mechanism Cymru in Wales. In Northern Ireland and Scotland there is no IRM. However, there are provisions for reviewing agency decisions about prospective carers.
3 NICE guidelines recommend consideration of bariatric surgery for BMI over 40, or over 35 with co-morbidities such as diabetes.

Given the other advantages offered by this couple, it would have been better practice for the following actions to have been undertaken.

- The medical adviser should have written to the applicants' general practitioner (copying the letter to Mr and Mrs W), requesting a review of their general health as part of their application. This should include ensuring that Mrs W has optimal control of her blood pressure, and Mr W optimal control of his diabetes. The general practitioner should have been asked to consider the NICE guidelines for the management of their obesity, which would include a referral for a specialist opinion about surgery, for example, gastric banding.[3]

- The social work report to the panel should then have addressed the following points:

  - What is the applicants' insight into the causes of their obesity and diabetes and how these problems can lead to long-term health impairment?

  - What is the applicants' understanding of a healthy diet for their family? Are their birth children overweight or obese? Have previous foster children placed with these applicants gained excessive weight?

  - What is the prospective adopters' attitude to physical activity, both for themselves and any children placed with them? What is their capacity to engage in physical activity? Do they become breathless climbing one flight of stairs? Could they chase a challenging child who runs towards a road? Are these applicants able to provide a young child with at least 60 minutes or more of physical activity every day?

  - Do the applicants want to lose weight? Successful weight loss depends very largely on motivation. An unmotivated applicant is unlikely to lose weight. Their previous history of successful and unsuccessful weight loss attempts is important.

  - Do the applicants have the time and/or resources to achieve successful weight loss?

- The local authority should then have assessed at the matching panel how they could support this placement, given the increased health risks, for example, leisure passes for the whole family, specialist physical activity for disabled children, respite care when adults require hospital admission for surgery, etc.

- The panel would then have had the opportunity to make a more balanced decision, taking all of the above factors into account. The serious health risks would then have been weighed against the fact that the little boy was very unlikely to find another adoptive family.

These actions would have saved the agency the costs of an IRM referral – money which could have been used to support the placement. Robust contingency planning for adverse health outcomes would have been more appropriate than entrenched views about potential health risk.

3. A foster carer who wishes to adopt

What are the issues involved in leaving a child in a placement which is apparently unhealthy, and how can health and social services work effectively together in the interests of the child?

Mrs P is a 49-year-old white, short-term foster carer who has been looking after Nicola, a 12-year-old white girl, for over two years. The local authority plan was for long-term fostering for Nicola, but there has been a considerable delay in identifying a suitable family. Mrs P has now put in an application to become Nicola's adoptive parent.

Mrs P has always been a cigarette smoker. Her last health assessment was two years ago. At that time, her BMI was 38 and she was not diabetic. Using the QRISK®2-2010 risk assessment tool, her risk of developing heart disease during the next 10 years was then 4 per cent. The new health assessment carried out as part of her adoption application assessment shows that Mrs P now has a BMI of 42. She is also a newly diagnosed diabetic. She is not hypertensive. Using the QRISK®2-2010 tool, her risk of developing heart disease during the next 10 years is 11 per cent. If she stops smoking, this risk will fall to 6 per cent. It would be useful for the medical adviser to discuss with the general practitioner whether Mrs P sticks to her diabetic diet, whether she attends the diabetic clinic follow-up appointments and whether she has been offered smoking cessation advice.

The medical adviser requests further information about Nicola from the looked after children's (LAC) nurse and/or school nurse. At her last review health assessment, the nurse was quite concerned about

Nicola. She was finding it very difficult to settle at secondary school, had gained a considerable amount of weight in the preceding 12 months and was alleging being bullied about her weight. She had recently started to refuse to go to school, especially on days when she had games or swimming.

On discussion with the fostering team, it becomes apparent that Mrs P did not think that either her own or Nicola's weight was a problem. Mrs P said that she had always had a heavy build and became quite angry during the discussion with the social worker. Mrs P had apparently tried numerous diets which had never worked. She thought that Nicola had "puppy fat" which she would outgrow. Mrs P thought it was unkind to restrict Nicola's access to sweets and cakes because of the difficult life she had led prior to coming into care. Mrs P saw nothing wrong with writing sick notes for Nicola on days when she had physical education.

A meeting of professionals should be called before the application is progressed, and the following people should be invited:

- the child's social worker;
- the foster carer link worker;
- the LAC nurse;
- the school nurse;
- the medical adviser to the adoption panel;
- the Head of Year at Nicola's secondary school.

The following issues should be considered at this meeting.

- What is the physical build of members of Nicola's birth family, i.e. her genetic build?
- Does the child have an unhealthy diet?
- Does she take adequate exercise? If not, is there another form of exercise that she might enjoy, for example, dancing?
- Are her eating patterns associated with low self-esteem?
- Is she "comfort" eating?
- What is her family background, for example, did she come from a family where there was significant neglect? Did she often go without food?
- Are there any other concerns about the placement apart from Nicola's weight? Have

other children in this placement gained weight?

- What can be done to support Nicola at home and at school?

- What can be done to change Mrs P's attitude to the problem and then to support her in changing her behaviour?

At this meeting, the medical adviser's role is to stress the importance of Mrs P stopping smoking, having good diabetic control and reducing her weight, to lower the chances of future serious health complications.

This information will take time to collect and will involve a number of further discussions with other colleagues. Two issues are in danger of being confused in this situation: firstly, the possible child protection issues in the current placement; and secondly, the adoption application.

Child protection can be defined as the process of protecting children from abuse or neglect, working to prevent impairment of their health and development, and making sure that they can grow up in circumstances consistent with the provision of safe, effective care which will allow them to develop to their full potential and enter adulthood successfully.

The child protection issues must be given priority. Any future discussion needs to be absolutely focused, thoroughly documented and must clearly differentiate between the two issues. It is absolutely essential to obtain Nicola's views of her placement and her understanding of the professionals' concerns.

There is a risk in leaving a vulnerable adolescent in an unhealthy environment, but is this a serious enough issue to require that the young person be removed? What are the grounds for any removal? Is the risk of Nicola staying where she is greater than the trauma of a placement move and a possible change of school?

Given the length of time Nicola has been in this placement, her foster carer could always make a direct application to court if she was not supported by the local authority, preventing any removal of the child.

Ultimately, any decisions will be made by social services/children's services. However, the recommendations of a multi-agency professionals' meeting and a rigorous problem-solving approach should lead to a balanced decision which is more transparent and more resistant to external challenge and scrutiny.

8   Conclusion

Medical advisers, social workers and panels will. continue to struggle with assessment of obesity in adult applicants because they are working in an area where there is little evidence-based research to support decision making. It is our hope that this guide will introduce some consistency of practice and encourage research in this area.

Obese adults are known to be at increased risk of significant health problems. These problems increase as obesity increases, and are made much worse when secondary complications develop. Obese children are at risk of increased health problems and are at increased risk of becoming obese adults.

Health and social services departments have a responsibility to ensure the health and welleing of children in care and their carers. Hence, they have a responsibility to identify and address obesity in substitute carers and in children and young people in the care system.

Children in care deserve the best environment we can give them, and starting to address the risks of obesity in their carers and themselves will help to give them an improved future, both physically and emotionally. Addressing obesity may be one of the most important things that any adult or child can do to protect their health and increase their life expectancy.

Every applicant and every child is unique. Both deserve holistic and comprehensive assessments of their individual circumstances. Hard and fast rules, in the absence of evidence, will prevent children finding the families they need.

Bibliography

Baumer HJ (2007) 'Obesity and overweight: its prevention, identification, assessment and management', *Archives of Disease in Childhood Education and Practice edition*, 92:3, pp 92–96

British Cardiac Society, British Hyperlipidaemia Association, British Hypertension Society and British Diabetic Association (2000) 'Joint British recommendations on the prevention of coronary heart disease in clinical practice: summary', *British Medical Journal*, 320, pp 705–08

British Heart Foundation (2010) Statistics website, available at: www.heartstats.org

Craig R, Mindell J and Hirani V (2009) *Health Survey for England 2008: Physical activity and fitness*, London: NHS Information Centre, available at: www.ic.nhs.uk/statistics-and-data-collections/health-and-lifestyles-related-surveys/health-survey-for-england/health-survey-for-england--2008-physical-activity-and-fitness

Cross-Government Obesity Unit, Department of Health and Department for Children, Schools and Families (2009) *Healthy Weight, Healthy Lives: A Cross-government strategy for England*, London: HM Government

Department for Children, Schools and Families and Department of Health (2007) *Looked After Children: We can and must do better*, London: DCSF and DH

Department for Children, Schools and Families and Department of Health (2009) *Promoting the Health and Well Being of Looked after Children* statutory guidance, London: DCSF and DH

Department for Education and Skills (2003) *Every Child Matters*, Green Paper, London: DfES

Department for Education and Skills (2006) *Care Matters: Transforming the lives of children and young people in care*, London: DfES

Department of Health (2002) *National Minimum Standards, Fostering Services Regulations (England)*, London: DH

Department of Health (2004) *At Least Five a Week: Evidence on the impact of physical activity and its relationship to health*, Report of the Chief Medical Officer, London: DH

Department of Health (2009) *UK-WHO Growth Charts*, available at www. growthcharts.rcpch.ac.uk

Department of Health and Children (1999) *National Standards for Foster Care*, Belfast, Department for Health and Children

Department of Health and Children (2009) *Health of the Population*, Belfast: Department of Health and Children, available at: www.dohc.ie/statistics/key_trends_2009/health_of_the_population/intro_2.html

Department of Health and Department for Children, Schools and Families (2008) *National Child Measurement Programme*, available at www.ic.nhs.uk/webfiles/publications/ncmp/ncmp0607/NCMP%202006%2007.%20Bulletin.pdf

Department of Health, Home Office, Department for Education and Skills and Department for Culture, Media and Sport (2007) *Safe. Sensible. Social: The next steps in the National Alcohol Strategy*, London: HM Government

Department of Health, Social Services and Public Safety (2007) *Care Matters: A bridge to a better future*, Belfast, DHSSPS

Després J-P, Lemieux I and Prud'Homme D (2001) 'Treatment of obesity: need to focus on high risk abdominally obese patients', *British Medical Journal*, 322, pp 716–20

Foresight (2007) *Tackling Obesities: Future Choices*, London: Government Offices for Science, available at www.foresight.gov.uk/

Hunt J, Waterhouse S and Lutman E (2008) *Keeping Them in the Family: Outcomes for children placed in kinship care through care proceedings*, London: BAAF

Jackson R (2000) 'New Zealand cardiovascular disease risk benefit prediction guide', *British Medical Journal*, 320, pp 709–10

Lindsay P and Hill C (2002) 'Objective assessment of vascular disease risk in prospective adoptive parents', *Adoption & Fostering*, 26:1, pp 74–76

National Heart, Lung and Blood Institute (1998) *Clinical Guidelines on Identification, Evaluation and Treatment of Overweight and Obesity in Adults: The evidence report*, Bethesda, MD: National Institutes of Health

National Institute of Clinical Excellence (2006) *Obesity: Guidance on the prevention, identification, assessment and management of overweight and obesity in adults and children*, Clinical Guideline 43, London: NICE

NHS (2004) General Medical Services Contract, London: NHS

NHS National Services Scotland (2009) *Obesity*, Edinburgh: NHS National Services Scotland, available at: www.isd.scot.nhs.uk/isd/5108.html

Rees R, Oliver K, Woodman J and Thomas J (2009) *Children's Views about Obesity, Body Size, Shape and Weight: A systematic review*, London: EPPI Centre, Social Science research unit, Institute of Education, London University, available at http://eppi.ioe.ac.uk/cms/Default.aspx?tabid=2466&language=en-US

Reilly JJ and Wilson D (2006) 'ABC of obesity: childhood obesity', *British Medical Journal*, 333, pp 1207–1210

Scottish Executive (2005) National Care Standards Foster Care and Family Placement Services, Edinburgh: Scottish Executive

Scottish Executive (2007) *Looked After Children and Young People: We can and must do better*, Edinburgh: Scottish Executive

Stunkard A, Thorkild I, Sorensen D, Hanis C, Teasdale T, Chakraborty R, Schull W and Schulsinger F (1986) 'An adoption study of human obesity', *New England Journal of Medicine*, 314, pp 193–198

Wake M, Hardy P, Sawyer MG and Carlin JB (2008) 'Comorbidities of overweight/obesity in Australian preschoolers: a cross sectional population study', *Archives of Disease in Childhood*, 93, pp 502–507

Warman A (2009) *Recipes for Fostering*, London: BAAF

Welsh Assembly Government (2003) *National Minimum Standards for Fostering Services (Wales)*, Cardiff: Welsh Assembly Government

Welsh Assembly Government (2004) *Children and Young People: Rights to Action*, Cardiff: Welsh Assembly Government

Whitaker RC, Wright JA, Pepe MS, Seidel K and Dietz W (1997) 'Predicting obesity in young adulthood from childhood and parental obesity', *New England Journal of Medicine*, 337, pp 869–730